HOMEOPATHY
Nature's Boon or an **Obsolete Myth**

SOMESH MADAN

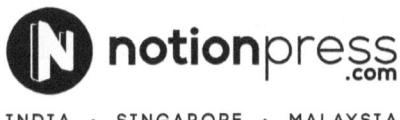

INDIA • SINGAPORE • MALAYSIA

Notion Press

No. 8, 3rd Cross Street,
CIT Colony, Mylapore,
Chennai, Tamil Nadu – 600 004

First Published by Notion Press 2020
Copyright © Somesh Madan 2020
All Rights Reserved.

ISBN 978-1-63606-743-8

This book has been published with all efforts taken to make the material error-free after the consent of the author. However, the author and the publisher do not assume and hereby disclaim any liability to any party for any loss, damage, or disruption caused by errors or omissions, whether such errors or omissions result from negligence, accident, or any other cause.

While every effort has been made to avoid any mistake or omission, this publication is being sold on the condition and understanding that neither the author nor the publishers or printers would be liable in any manner to any person by reason of any mistake or omission in this publication or for any action taken or omitted to be taken or advice rendered or accepted on the basis of this work. For any defect in printing or binding the publishers will be liable only to replace the defective copy by another copy of this work then available.

Disclaimer

The content of this book is for informational purposes only and is not intended to diagnose, treat or cure any condition or disease. The reader understands that this book is not intended as a substitute for consultation with a licensed practitioner. The reader should regularly consult a physician in matters relating to his/her health and particularly with respect to any symptoms that may require diagnosis or medical attention. Any characters, events and incidents mentioned in the illustrations are either the products of the author's imagination or used in a fictitious manner. Any resemblance to actual persons, living or dead, or actual events is purely coincidental. The use of this book implies your acceptance of this disclaimer.

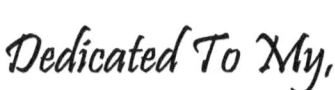

Dedicated To My,

Father,
for giving me the best of everything in life

my **Mother**,
for always encouraging my ventures

my **Brother**,
for being an original classic

my **Wife, Lyudmila,**
for showing me dreams can become a reality.

There are no words that will ever do justice to how grateful I am to have you in my life.

and off course

to my curious reader out there:
may you find happiness

in good health

Contents

Preface *11*

1. The Immunity Chakra. 13
2. The Modern Ghazi 19
3. The Viral Affaire' .25
4. The Endless Pursuit 31
5. The Misshapen Destiny 39
6. The Vocal Pacifier 57
7. The Alpha Legacy 67

Preface

Through this book I hope to enlighten those people who solidify their facts about Homeopathy based on few failed attempts or misconceptions. More importantly, this book will help you in understanding Homeopathy as well as your body much better. The book will reward you with the power to choose and make your own decisions to live a healthier life not just in the present, but the future as well!

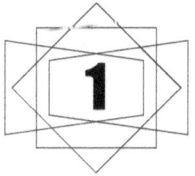

The Immunity Chakra

"What a brilliant day it is to be alive", I exclaimed. The day was Friday, the 13th of May 1994 and there was nothing superstitious about it in the mind of a six year who was relieved to be done with school for the summer. Summers can be testing in India with temperatures going well over a hundred degrees Fahrenheit, but it's the *season of mangoes* and everyone looks forward to its arrival.

As a child I was no different than any other brat who wanted his share of fun. That meant the day

I could save 10 Rupees (equivalent to 50 Rupees today) after school to spend on canteen was a lottery for me. Now wait a second, let's rewind back the clocks a bit so we don't mistake me to be a deprived child tied to chains at home. My childhood is filled with memories of my father who always managed to take out time to spoil me while working as a Senior ENT Surgeon travelling abroad. Never did he raise his hand on me or scold me, though my mother would never agree with that. She came from her own family of disciplinarians and was a Teacher for all the right reasons. At that age I thought I had cracked the code at getting away with anything by just being on my best behavior whenever my folks were around. How juvenile of me.

One might think this is every child's life, why write about it? That is correct and that is the mistake most people commit about Homeopathy without getting in depth to understand the psychology of the patient and the inception of the symptoms the first time. Growing up between a doctor and a teacher, I was not allowed to have cold drinks or soda pop, all sorts of candy was banned and pets were frowned upon as the cause of all the allergies you can find in our world. The world my parents had created was practical, loving but with a hint of paranoia over diseases. Fast forward to Friday, May 13th 1994 and now you would understand why I was overjoyed as a child to be able to earn my allowance to discreetly have a Coke. I would be lying if I said I did not enjoy it. At home there were no burgers or pizzas or any junk food ever and I remember whatever new thing we tried was from our mother's kitchen when she tirelessly cooked for us from scratch or for a friend's birthday party. A sneeze may mean in a normal household as a sign to offer someone a tissue but in our house it meant a dose of Homeopathy, *Aconitum* namely and an interrogation to find the cause. This is one of the major reasons while most children enjoyed eating outside way more with their parents, I would mostly hide to do the same. It took me quite a few years to understand my rebellious nature and also my fondness for all animals. Over the last few decades I met several people who blamed my father's over protective nature for my weak immunity compared to others and I'm sure there are many others who would attribute it to the same reason.

Indeed I regret not being born in Punjab in the fresh open farms where every day I got a glass of creamy lassi[1] and a giant parantha[2] with a scoop of butter because nothing beats a good diet. It may not be balanced to perfection and it may not be always healthy but it is something each one of us forgets to pay attention over time. So instead of dwelling on the past the next time I felt flu or viral, instead of rushing to take a Homeopathic or an Allopathic medicine, I simply gargled with salt water and used nature's remedies. Over time I noticed there were moments where I had to take a medicine when the situation worsened but seven out of ten times I managed to get well without any prescription drugs. Grownups I feel live in a more complicated world than children and several tricks are thrown around to improve our immunity whether it is taking Probiotic capsules each day, drinking Aloe Vera in the morning and so on. The fact of the matter is that the reader should listen to me not because I am no longer a child but because I have tried these methods over a given period of time and also witnessed the effect on others before sharing them here.

---

[1] a sweet Indian drink made from yogurt or buttermilk.
[2] flattened bread.

No amount of probiotic ammunizers can save us entirely from falling sick if someone around us has a flu or has been coughing or sneezing the entire day. No amount of drinking healthy liquids and plant extracts can guarantee us 100% immunity, period. Basically all these are meant to build the body's immunity but it's shocking to discover that every person has a different benefit level from such ammunizers, though most benefits are negligible to even notice. In the end, I wouldn't like to conclude by taking us all on a ride and leaving mid-way saying the morale here is to eat healthy and stay alert. The revelation here is to not assume eating junk food is always bad, it is extremely important to enjoy the moments and make the most of it. It is surprising how many well built people are vulnerable to falling ill. It comes as a shock to our world today if a 6 feet 3 inch man weighing over 230 pounds dies of a heart attack suddenly but if an average man who weighs 140 pounds falls ill, it will not surprise anyone. Unfortunately people forget – looking fit & being fit are two very different things!

But Homeopathy has no role in building one's immunity and if anything I learnt, it was that the more often we take Homeopathy for the little things, more prone we become to falling prey again. On the other hand if we take refuge in Homeopathy at the first sign or symptom, it can save us a big deal of trouble but we won't get into that until later.

For an immunity that lasts as long as the Queen of England, it is essential to understand the body first and foremost. Listen to the signs and don't take any symptom or medicine for granted. It's good to have the necessary vitamins but it's even better to get a regular blood test to know exactly what our body requires and then consume it. Most importantly, go for a workout no matter how trivial or hardcore it maybe and eat right. Eating at odd hours and food that's not cooked in our kitchen is one of the main reasons we can never be entirely sure of the *thief*.

The Immunity Chakra has for decades confused everyone with different theories emerging every new day, but not anymore. Not you!

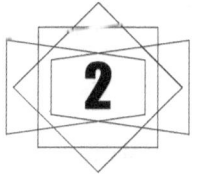

The Modern Ghazi

Is the human body capable of healing itself infinite times?

There is no secret to that, only ignorance.

We have all experienced pain at some point in our lives, whether it was a childhood injury, a sports injury trying to have fun as a grown up or just surviving life in today's time.

As a naïve brat, I myself garnished scars on each limb but wouldn't go as far as to say I loved getting them. Being a football fanatic, I would find my ankle twisted often apart from the mundane gashes here and there. The sprain & twisted ankles would be then addressed by my mother's ancient homemade remedies which included turmeric in warm milk and hot bandages.

While my new injury would create a mini tsunami in our small home, my father would sneakily escape the chaos to return with *Arnica* and *Hypericum* – two homeopathic medicines, which would become a beacon during my darkest moments. Over the years I grew to face such situations many a times, where without Homeopathic medicines I was forced to take painkillers. They were called *magic pills* where you took one and the relief was immediately effective. It made so much sense why everyone in the world preferred popping a pill rather than wait for a Homeopathic medicine to take its precious time, a few hours to be precise, to give relief. But that's where I was ignorant, for believing in something solely because the world does.

Arnica and *Hypericum* have been long known as the natural Homeopathic remedies for treatment of swelling, pain and bleeding. So after using a gym for three years while being trained by their non-certified instructor, it came as no surprise to me when my shoulder injury became a constant muscle pain. The break from the gym fixed things but only till I kept lying in bed like an Egyptian mummy. "No problem, I have magic pills in my drawer!" I exclaimed to myself happily. But here's the bemusing fact with most common painkillers people realize over time – the relief is temporary and usually wears off in twelve hours. No way forgetting, the massive list of *sneaky* side-effects they carry which can be found much easily on the Internet now, than in 2005. Like the reader, I too was no special and ignored most of these side-effects till one of them actually surfaced and made me realize the gravity of the situation.

In 2009 when I suffered a shooting pain in the neck which left me immobile, I took charge of the situation having woken up to the fact that painkillers are not a long lasting treatment. In simple words, I was just delaying the process with temporary relief and with a sign of helplessness knowing the pain will eventually return. Some people wander their whole life suffering, their whole life looking for a realistic permanent cure but not knowing whether there really is a way out. After using Homeopathic medicines such as *Arnica* and *Hypericum*, for well over two decades, I tried to decipher how these paradoxes work. Taking a high potency of these medicines would not guarantee a quicker relief, but the **right potency** at the **right time** can change our world. In fact the selection of potency is the most crucial stage and dogmatic instructions simply don't work here. The relief with Homeopathy is not sudden but gradual which one would realize probably after the second dose or two hours, but even this delay gives an extended sense of satisfaction as we feel the relief and realize this is a lasting cure. Homeopathy doesn't just temporarily pause the suffering but in fact provides a cure, while treating the root cause over a period of time.

"How can you wait so long to feel better?" many would ask me without much conviction until now.

"Well, simply because when the pain or swelling subsided after taking homeopathic medicines, it was a permanent relief. Not just for 12 hours or with side effects", I would confidently say.

Human are strange creatures and we often make mistakes forgetting we are mortals. But to not learn from those mistakes is an even graver one. Over the years our body's self-healing properties slowly diminish and the lifestyle plays its role in harbouring other poisonous ailments. There are many amongst us who play this brilliant role of masking their injuries or pretend to be oblivious towards the hardening truth. They play this role flawlessly when visiting a dozen physicians, a couple of other physiotherapists and a few acupuncture sessions even. All while masking a smile that hides their grim hope that their injury or muscle pain will perhaps disappear forever today. Humans are strange creatures indeed.

We have a relentless hope inside us that makes us believe where there is darkness, there will be light. Yet we never choose to do things differently than others. So how can this darkness turn into light? After being such a creature myself, I learnt with time how to carefully listen to my body when it spoke to me and at times even without saying when it needed me. Homeopathy was the last option for me after countless failed treatments had led me back to where I began. It was then I realized that the most long-lasting relief I got in the world was after taking *Arnica* and *Hypericum.* Indeed "Warriors" in the world of Homeopathy is what I would call them as they do not just reduce the swelling and the unbearable pain but also definitely speed up the process of healing. When one understands the possibilities Homeopathy has to offer without affecting our health in a negative manner, we realize really which one are the *magic pills* really!

In today's world the most priceless gift you can give someone is – time. We are all short of it and wish the day was more than just twenty four hours. For our family, time was a matter of perspective. The most priceless gift my father taught me we could have in life is good health, without which time itself would not hold much meaning.

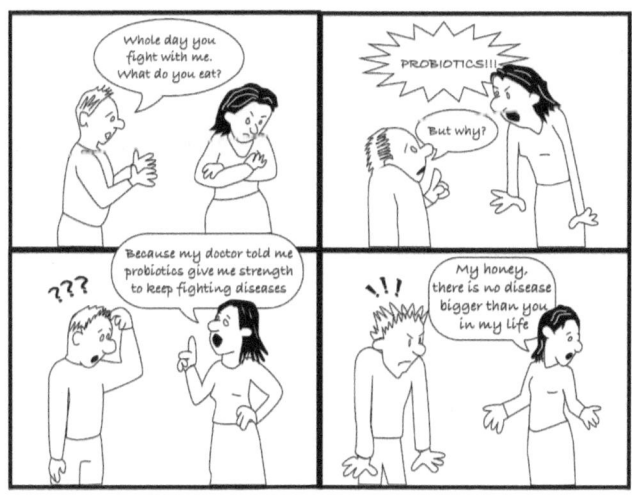

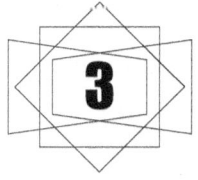

3

The Viral Affaire'

The setting is perfect.

Those gorgeous monsoon days where the sun plays hide and seek and everyone in India finds some relief from the sweltering heat is not at all an uncommon sight.

There is not much difference between children and grownups, for we all have moments in life where we mentally time travel to our past or our future self. As a child we used to love getting drenched in the rain and while most children were not allowed to step out, courtesy of their over protective parents, we would make most of every joy we could steal in this world before apple became more than just a fruit.

In the 1990's air conditioners were still a dream many middle class families in India were realizing and a much needed one considering India can see temperatures glare to overwhelming heights. I would later realize those over protective parents were not entirely dense, since catching a cold during rainy season was a common in those days. To add to this peril, the air conditioning itself was a catalyst which fluctuated our body temperatures as we ran in and out of rooms. It is a very different phenomenon till date for many foreigners who are used to central air conditioning and have never come across it.

The life of a child in his mind is often without a purpose. Until he realizes that every decision of his influences the person he becomes tomorrow.

The episode would start with a harmless sneeze and before I could contemplate who took off my wet clothes from the rain, my father would have already given me *Aconitum*. The power of this Homeopathic medicine was inevitable to ignore through all stages of my life, as I was yet to learn.

The next day the story would unfold as we friends would all meet as seven year olds ready to invent a new game, but few were missing. While some would still have a runny nose, there was always that one guy who got fever because of the temperature change. "Well, unlucky him", we used to think hoping our friend would be better soon. For some of my readers, this chapter would feel like a sincere waste of time and I don't blame you for feeling that. Most of us would think the human body is indeed capable of taking care of a cold itself, when the truth actually is far from it.

Like a virus true to its name, it comes in many forms, names and symptoms that are all still not know to humans. There are some of us who have a slightly stronger immunity than the rest, *Gold Class* as we would refer to them. The *Gold Class* patients can afford a cold and running nose for months without developing any other symptoms. Eventually they succumb to nasal drops and anti allergy pills which are prescribed, without realizing that it soon becomes a part of their daily lives. The cold eventually does go away but not entirely as the antihistamines only temporary cool the situation down. The infection which has now been masked as an allergy then continues to grow while being dormant, only to re-appear in the form of sinus in most patients. Like many of us, this situation is a never ending loop which gives the illusion that there is a cure in the end when there is not. Not without Homeopathy getting involved.

Then there are also those of us who suffer the usual weather changing symptoms, the virus morphing itself in the form of bone chills, fever and extreme weakness. I would call us the *Silver Class*, for we truly understand how worse a cold can get. Most of us experience such symptoms without realizing where it all began and how will it all ends. Could this situation be controlled if we took *Aconitum* when we first sneezed?

The answer is most certainly – yes. Over the past two decades, I have come across people who have been bonafide as well as malifide speakers for Homeopathy. In my own family I witness those who label Homeopathy as being nothing more than a mad science experiment and then there are people who have willingly tried it for the sole purpose of a safer treatment. Fortunately for the latter, Homeopathy has shown brilliant results if taken as a preventive measure in most cases. I am certain there are those in the world who will argue as to why should we administer any medicine (even if Homeopathy) before actually confirming serious symptoms. To them my befitting reply should be transparent; as I am not aiming to encourage any reader here to put more faith in taking a medicine each time anything happens. I ask you to put your faith in knowing your own body more closely. When you can read the signs your body gives you, over time it can help you predict symptoms before letting them overpower you. Our childhood is most fun we ever have our whole lives, but it is the time between our past and now that teaches us how to care better for our body in future. As a child I've met children whose parents never paid attention to such things and eventually they would need a sinus surgery when they were just eighteen. By the time I was an adult, I noticed how common it is to just take an antihistamine for a cold and forget about it for the rest of the day. Well until, the infection returned in the form of sinus as I mentioned earlier, with different triggering symptoms such as migraines and ringing of the ears.

Is it not peculiar how we behave casual about the things that may affect oneself in the course of time inevitably? We make our ignorance into a reality and survive on that till it is no longer possible.

Most of us are too simple to connect the dots, but it is all connected. Even today after more than thirty years I would hope our position with fighting such viruses would become better but we are far from it. Not just in India but all over the world, every year people face such symptoms and blame it on the season or on a virus which is *just in the air nowadays*. They seem to have accepted their fate it seems, but hopefully not you. Homeopathic marvels in today's time such as *Aconitum*, if taken on the first sign of a symptom have proven time and again to be an armour without any hidden baggage.

As my father would make his point clear to us as children, "It is not important how strong a medicine is that we take, or how fast it gives us relief alone. What truly matters is how safe that medicine is to our body in the long run."

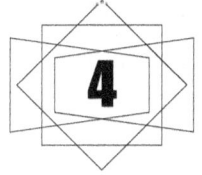

The Endless Pursuit

A human is genetically designed to experience three stages in life.

The first stage of life is when self-consciousness awakens, the second stage, when self-realization awakens and the last, the self-improvement stage.

All throughout their lives, humans are consistently trying to create a better version of themselves. Through this relentless yet constant pursuit, there are many of us who fall prey to skin infections and encounter sufferings which can be quite personal at times to be discussed openly.

Let us address the elephant in the room today, shall we?

"10 minutes more Mom, I'll be home soon I promise", the nine year old me would exclaim, counting every minute out of the house as – *a good minute.* Being raised by two strict academic parents, as a child I took my playtime very seriously. I was good at sports and even better at inventing new games which me and my friends would profusely enjoy playing, losing all track of time. Just like any child at my age would perhaps, I had the victorious scars to prove how much fun we had, until my mother would catch up to my charade and drag me home. When we grew up we realized how exotic it is to be in countries with tropical climates but also realized that it was inevitable to not sweat. That isn't a bad sign actually as many would worry if their child sweats too much, but recent scientific research has shown us that it is completely normal.

But sweating profusely time and again taught me there is a bigger issue at stake here than everything else – *the elephant in the room* – Fungal & Bacterial infections.

On an average I would speak (solely based on my interaction with others) that almost every person suffers a bacterial or fungal infection at some point in their life. This can be due to excessive sweating, compromised immune system or simply a bad hygiene regime. Unfortunately the ironic part of this infection is its physical appearance which deters many to share their suffering, even when most of them have experienced it and felt isolated. Fungal and Bacterial infections are notorious for re-occurring and are generally treated with strong antibiotics that control the extent as it spreads like wildfire.

When we were in school my father used to proudly share with me how his meticulously researched Acne Homeopathic formula worked on a student from my class. My father has for decades observed the side effects of strong allopathic pills and unnecessary medications, having lost his own brother at an age when he did not know much about the safe treatment techniques offered with Homeopathy. When you see a light at the end of the tunnel, it is bound to bring a smile on your face.

During the same time, it was summers and I was busier than usual practicing to get into my school football team and in the evenings, be practicing again for a local badminton tournament that was going to take place. By the time it was evening and

I was drenched in sweat, I caught my breath on reaching home before jumping in the shower to cool down. During this time, I suddenly felt a slight itch on my thigh and though it was still young, I could see the circular region it was making. With worried eyes I showed it to my father to attempt to understand what we were dealing with here. But it did not take my father long to diagnose that it was a fungal infection and I should take homeopathy and wait. Bad decision! The next day when I woke up, the itching had spread and was much more severe. Clearly the infection had more power and homeopathy was unable to catch up to its speed at which it was growing.

How can you tell a genuine doctor from an incompetent one? A genuine doctor will never hesitate to admit if one diagnosis of theirs does not work and swiftly make changes in their treatment rather than letting the patient suffer to guard one's own ego. I realize this genuine quality came to my father through decades of experience treating patients of all kinds as he immediately decided that morning to start me on a stronger fungal medicine, an allopathic course for five days. I was apprehensive and uncomfortable having seen the magnitude at which this fungal infection was spreading covering most of my thigh in one day itself. But taking the allopathic medicine indeed helped as the next day I could notice the severity of the itch decrease and the infection had not spread to new areas. Still shocked but grateful to my father for choosing this option, he explained me very calmly, "It is very essential to judge the stage of infection you are dealing with because Homeopathy does not help if the infection is at a later stage or very severe. If the infection you feel has taken a serious turn for the worse, it is always advisable to take a stronger medicine. But in cases when the infection is still at an early stage, Homeopathy shows promising results."

I have never forgotten what he told me that day. There are so many people in today's world that face fungal infections whether it is in their private regions in the form of an itch, on their feet in the form of an unpleasant odour (long hours wearing shoes) or even on toe-nails due to bad hygiene. The same way bacterial infections have given a stiff competition for they too can spread at a rapid speed. We all have that one person in our lives who likes to burst their pimple or just scratch it the minute they realize its existence. The bitter truth is that this actually is the best recipe to spread the infection, but I am sure everyone in today's time knows that but somehow just can't resist not caring at times.

Human has always been contemplating the concept of good health. The main reason for that is the shortage of time itself in today's world. Instead of trying to perceive good health, what if you could attain it in a simpler way?

What my father told me that day made me question myself, "What if we mix the good elements of both the worlds and diagnose the situation timely?" The self-realization stage has awoken indeed.

With that my whole idea of dealing with this situation changed. In the process I learnt that Homeopathic powders such as *Borodula*, when applied to a suspected area help prevent this situation from ever arising. Also, the Homeopathic medicine *Acid Nitricum* is an unexpected treasure that works effectively in early stages of such skin disorders and infections. There is truth about fungal and bacterial infections reoccurring in more than half of its patients but paying more attention has confirmed this chain can be broken indeed. But regularly maintaining a self hygiene is tragically not enough in today's time. Most patients forget the most basic rule of the human body – we are what we eat. And those who have a sweet tooth (or teeth) are always more prone to developing fungal infections as it misbalances our body's primary constitution and encourages the growth.

I would suggest every patient out there who feels this is a relentless infection which keeps coming back to try these methods and not lose hope. You my reader are not alone in this world!

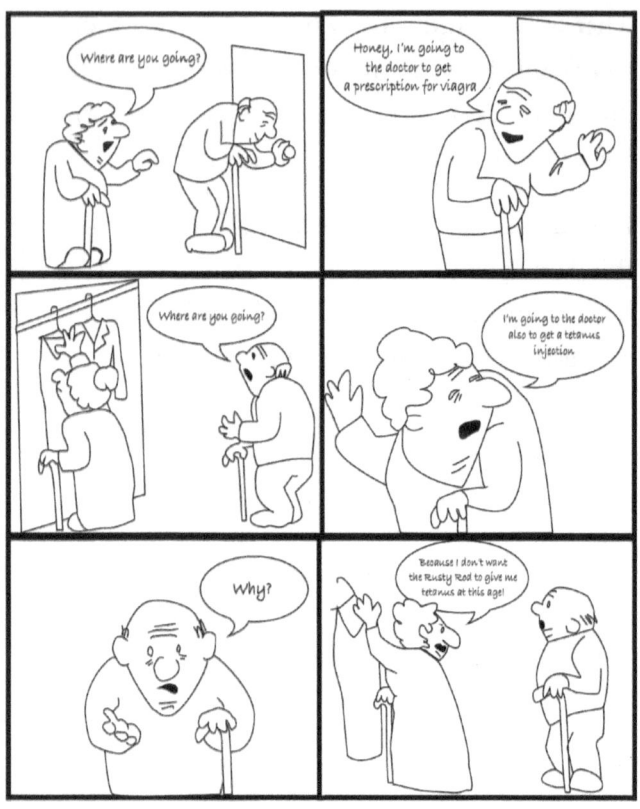

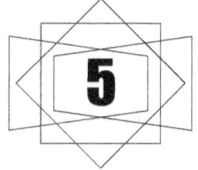

The Misshapen Destiny

The beginning of the end or the end of the beginning.

Which moment really determines that? Until it is staring at us deep in our eyes.

When we are young, we all have our guilty pleasures we would not think twice to sin for. Out of all of the simple bliss life has to offer, children enjoy gorging on outside food the most. That longing in their eyes and a desire to get a break from mom's kitchen is something every parent has witnessed.

"Birthday party? Oh yes!"

I jumped with joy as probably a hundred chocolates burst in my heart creating oodles of happiness. Then I went to my room and started planning what gift my friend would like and what all we will get to eat. Like most parents dutifully, I was not allowed to eat junk food from outside. While my friends were allowed to eat seldom still, I was allowed a treat only once a month leaving me high and dry the remaining twenty nine days.

Hence birthday parties were a heaven filled with treasure troves of pizzas, burgers, cakes, cold drinks and the lots. It was a huge success as my parents were not there to keep an eye on me and I truly felt like a Bond villain smirking to myself then. This happiness is not an exaggeration as my father being a doctor was genuinely more cautious than most parents were. By the time I was seventeen, I had memorized all the popular fast food joint's contact digits by heart. I am a foodie and like most Delhites felt there is nothing wrong in eating food that makes one feel happy. Healthy food is certainly inviting but I would enjoy a hot chocolate fudge any day over a vegan bowl of soup.

Just a few days after my twenty second birthday, I happen to notice an itch on my right leg which seemed to not be a mosquito bite or anything I had seen before. Since it was on my leg and not my face, it was never given the attention it should have been given and time moved on. By the time I was 24, I started facing inadmissible gastric issues every other night. It would start with extreme discomfort in the abdomen to severe acidity at times. But being my father's son I tried to access each time what could be the reason behind it. I noticed even eating at home gave me the same symptoms and I started putting it off to my bad timings and lifestyle being the catalyst here. Fast forward to four years after, I made sure to never travel anywhere in the world without an antacid in my baggage. Even when I travelled to Rome to enjoy my second true love – pizza, I was a pun of all jokes as my friends found my palpable collection of antacid medicines. Again, my father and I convinced myself it was because of my diet or the lifestyle that was causing this to happen. But as a patient I always sensed there was more than just that being a cause otherwise why it would suddenly be occurring at such an alarming frequency. By now we were adults and I would see so many people around me consuming antacids that I felt it wasn't just a big deal anymore. Well, slap my head and call me Judy because that's how naïve I was.

A few years ago, just days before my twenty eight birthday, I woke up with an itchy red spot on my leg. Blaming it on the confounded mosquitoes eager to taste my sweet blood, I itched and tried to get on with my day. The severity of the itch I soon realized was not normal as it persisted the entire day and continued to increase. The next morning when I woke up, the spot had become bigger and localized, looking more like an ant bite than a mosquito one. Afraid and concerned that it might be a fungal infection, even though it was an unlikely location for one, I took all the necessary precautions to eliminate any cause. I immediately made an appointment to see a skin specialist with my father who was fairly quick to prescribe an ointment and anti-bacterial pills. Unfortunately I got no result and hoped that like the itch I had faced on my leg several years ago, this might just disappear on its own as well. But after about ten days, two more itch spots appeared with the same burning severity that would make you want to peel your skin off. As I was travelling during this unfortunate discovery, I tried to behave normal even though I could feel that was going to take a lot from me. This wasn't just a mosquito bite or an allergy rash and not being able to understand what was wrong I visited our family skin specialist again who affirmed me it was a fungal infection and prescribed me even stronger medicines this time. Even though I knew these medicines had an adverse effect on the liver, I happily complied since I was tired of the continuous itchy spots by then. But how little did I know back then that this was all just the beginning to an end for me.

The medicine eventually ended up providing no relief so after three months of feeling helpless we decided to visit our family physician. After an observation lasting ten minutes, barely, his diagnose was scabies[3] and again I was prescribed strong medicines and a lotion to apply on my entire body to sleep in for two consecutive nights. It was dreadful to be covered in a lotion which smelt like chemicals and not even be sure if this would actually work. They say you never know what you are truly made of until you are faced by a peril where there is no coming back. This phase was truly one of the darkest phases of my life as not

---

[3] a type of skin infestation.

just Homeopathy, but any medication without a confirmed diagnose was turning out to be pointless. To add to my misery, the physical uneasiness of this situation was affecting my mental health and the uncertainty of the situation continued to make me more anti-social. I did get relief for a few hours or half a day but it was never long lasting enough to assure us. While my mother travelled abroad, she had no idea what my father and I were going through as we ransacked our entire apartment making sure every bed sheet, every cloth, in fact even the mattress was dry cleaned. Before we are all assumed to be paranoid lunatics, one must know this is the official protocol that has to be followed if a person is ever suspected to have scabies. One may think what the hell this scabies is and we've never heard of it before. I don't blame anyone for being ignorant, since I was on the same page and this was probably the exact time when I started researching more. Desperate to find out what's wrong with me I spent countless nights reading online forums about other patients who had shared their sufferings, facing similar symptoms as mine and spent a decade trying to make sense of it all. I was getting more and more anxious by the hour and my father could sense that as he tried to help me. But as a grownup, we all assume if we fall sick no matter what, at least we would have some medicine we can take to treat ourselves with. We rely on doctors and medicines to have a cure for everything that we will go through in this life.

But what if we or all the doctors around us can't figure out the cause itself? Would our decisions change if we realize life may never be the same again?

Going against my natural expectations, every new medicine made my relief even more short lived. The next day I would get random outbreaks of rash all over my body. The worst was that they would appear anywhere at anytime which made it harder for even day to day tasks to be completed by me. On behest of my worried father, I visited our physician once again who felt this was perhaps because of eating outside food too much and to quote exactly, advised me – "avoid chicken and meat". That was another kick below the belt for a non-vegetarian food lover to be told you can't eat out, but hold on, now you can't even eat meat cooked at your own house. Sigh!

But it had been more than six months and by now I would do anything to just get rid of this ailment.

I have considered myself a fairly hygiene conscious person throughout my life. I am not one of those lazy humans who fall asleep in their denims and have kept my standards intact even when I was travelling or eating outside. On top of all this, I had been a fashion model during my early college days and was quite proud of my flawless skin. Sure as a child we did eat tons of junk food, but who doesn't? I would convince myself to not panic, but when even doctors can't find what is wrong, you start looking for other sources to learn more about your symptoms. That is exactly what I did because any sort of physical skin ailment first and foremost starts alienating the patient from the world. The lonelier one gets with their thoughts, the faster their mental composure breaks down. All throughout this time I'm sure any mere mortal would just take an antihistamine and feel some comfort, even if it was for a temporary few hours.

But here's the truth that most doctors don't tell their patients and it ends up making them dependant on anti-allergy pills their whole life. An anti-allergy pill works by producing an antihistamine in your body that calms your allergy down for temporarily. Keep in mind, it is doing nothing to remedy the root cause and hence it is but natural that the symptoms will reappear. In the last two years I have come across several such patients in real life as well as on online medical forums who over time have become addicted to taking such antihistamines and whenever they try to stop or reduce it now, their allergy comes back way worse than before. In short, the medicine mankind gets the most relief and hopes from is nothing more than a delay in the real treatment itself. In the end, we can do whatever we wish to see sense in, but we cannot see what we can't make sense of yet.

Many people noticed my strong will when I never itched whether it was a pimple or a mosquito bite I got, not even as a child. But this itch was so severe that I have never felt it as intense before. Nonetheless, I may have been down but if fate had me to lose, I was going to give it a good fight anyhow. I decided not to take antihistamines merely because I did not want to mask the situation and wanted transparency to know what was really going on. The symptoms changed drastically as the itchy spots were just a teaser I realized. After a few days, I got a severe rash in the form of psoriasis on both my cheeks, which was then followed by random boils on my torso and outbreaks of hives even with no logical reason. It had been more than nine months that I was eating home food now and this crisis perplexed everyone. Our physician had no other option but to prescribe me another dose of the strong scabies medicine and it's a fact that has been branded well by our seniors – "He, who has still not found a cure for his suffering, will try anything before this unrest entirely consumes him."

Hence I complied having no other option what to do. But after all these months of stuffing myself with powerful medicines which had even stronger side effects, my body could not bear it anymore. In just two doses my digestive system was on fire and I got diarrohea which we found out was a common side effect of that medicine. The ironical fact was that I could sense this was not curing my real illness either. On top of that I was now an unwilling vegetarian, suffering with skin problems I had never had before and further being drained by digestive problems arising from the very medicine I took to cure me in the first place. By the time the longest twelve months of my life had crossed, I had accepted my fate that things would never be the same again. Eventually our physician gave up and my father could not find the culprit either. I distanced myself from my friends, since I could not eat outside nor wanted to be tempted by others who did. I would travel everywhere with an anti allergy pill in my wallet not knowing when I have a rash or worse. Then one fine day in the thirteenth month of this episode, I had a severe itchy spot which was more severe than the ones previously. "Relax, it's okay now you know the drill", I said as I tried to reassure my sinking heart. But spoke too soon I realized as this was nothing like I had ever witnessed before. The spot was bright red and in pairs so what I thought was just one, turned out to be four on one leg and two more on my hand. The itching would get worse in hot showers and during the nights. But in the daytime it would be bearable, though the spots kept increasing in size.

We can't fight death, but all that we face in our life before death is due to a cause and reaction. If you could find that cause & change your actions, would you still be making the same decisions as before?

By now I was reading various medical forums and trying to find answers to my symptoms. Pain and suffering that had lasted for more than a year while I was treated like an experiment was being replaced by reason and hope as I noticed there were many others who had faced my plight. After two days of carefully examining my spots growing, I noticed they were becoming filled with a yellow fluid inside them and when I put all my symptoms together, I found other sufferers online who had faced the exact same symptoms as I had all this while. The cause of this eventually turned out to be a severe *Gluten Allergy*.

One doesn't develop a gluten allergy at a certain given age to be precise. Most of those who have it would have been carrying it their entire lives. During our adolescence, our allergies get masked and appear with minute or admissible symptoms which make it harder to identify the true cause. Gluten, in easier words is the wheat component found in products such as roti[4], burger, pizza, cake and the list goes on. In fact in today's time most products have gluten present in them without us even realizing it. A brilliant example of such hidden gluten can be Sushi, which one would think is just fermented rice and stuffing of your kind but in reality there is a substance mixed in the sushi rice (holding it in shape) that is made purely of gluten. And because it is not deemed compulsory by the

---

[4] round flatbread native to India.

regulators, most brands & restaurants need not label their products or inform their customer as to whether they contain gluten or not. This however is changing now as more and more people wake up to trying a healthier eating lifestyle. Though over the years a gluten free diet has been advertised by many fitness enthusiasts, the reason for that is solely because gluten is actually a protein found in wheat and is not easily digestible by the human body even by those who are not allergic to it. Our body in fact struggles to digest gluten and it is primarily responsible for giving a food item its aesthetic definition. Once we understand how it works, it makes more sense as to why people who avoid gluten in their diet tend to find it makes a immense difference. But those who are allergic to it have to pay extra attention to avoid it, as I was going to learn firsthand myself.

When I first diagnosed myself after reading several online forums, I could not believe it. An Indian boy who has eaten roti all his life is now allergic to wheat? Life as they say my friend is not without a hint of irony. The realization that I could no longer eat pizzas and other things which were my favourite feel-good foods sent a shiver down my spine. But there was a sense of relief that came with this shiver as after more than a year of pointless suffering and senseless symptoms, all of this made sense. Once I graduated high school, all I had eaten was food which had mostly been a gluten full diet and had never been ashamed to admit that. Obviously when I shared this good news with my physician he was not too keen having never dealt with a patient with a gluten allergy before. As for me, I couldn't care less!

I informed my father what I had just found and shared with him that not only did all of my symptoms make sense but it was also highly possible why no other remedy worked on me all this time. Since I was eating breads and consuming gluten throughout this period without knowing this fact. But now the thief had been caught. When you know who the thief is, it is easy to corner and capture it. That is exactly what our plan was now. I immediately stopped all gluten from my diet which I would confess was not easy. It was still a time in India when not many people were aware of a gluten free diet and even less options were available to compensate for them. My diet changed from a couple of breads to rice and curry each day. It would be a blatant lie if I would remark the change in my diet made no difference, but the relief I got was immediately noticed as a blessing. The severity of my itching fell rapidly and no new spots or rashes erupted just out of the blue. Since we now knew the cause was an allergy, my father gave me a Homeopathic medicine *Natrum Mur* for it which further escalated my relief. This Homeopathic medicine has been well known for fighting allergies and with no life threatening side effects which I had faced before. But it is essential to pay attention the potency we take as taking the highest potency does not guarantee a faster relief. I took *Natrum Mur 1 Million* and felt my allergy get worst the first two days and then slowly subside. But when I was given *Natrum Mur* in a smaller potency such as 30 or 200, there was no aggravation and more relief that was immediately felt.

In this entire time, I visited doctors who were experts in their field, I took medicines which otherwise my father would never give me, but in the end what worked was me killing my own ignorance. It not only emerges from countless online researches but from understanding my body the best way that anyone can. I always encourage others to talk to someone and share their plight because you never know where in another corner of the world someone might have experienced the same symptoms as you.

There are indeed people in this world who come to amuse me with a constipated expression of shock on their faces when they ask me what a gluten free diet really means. Then there are those who get impressed by superficial beauty more than realistic facts and want to enquire from me how I keep fit when their life's sole purpose is to reduce weight. Does gluten free diet help keep you fit?

It sure does, which is one of the reasons it is also not an easy diet to follow unless you are allergic to it. Most people I come across can only manage to be on a gluten free diet for a few weeks before realizing they can't do it. Fortunately those who are allergic don't have that option and just like me have realized how a gluten free diet not just helps those allergic but in several other ways.

Since I have gone gluten free, I have felt my skin get better and less sensitive the way it first was during my college days. I don't have skin abnormalities in the form of what I have been through before. But what surprised me more than anything was my gastric issue getting resolved on its own. In five years of my life I realized I did not need any antacid anymore and never felt any discomfort in my stomach again. Everything that was happening to me was solely because of a diet which my body was no longer accepting. Sadly, there are still so many people in the world who face such digestive discomforts, skin infections or other symptoms and they or their doctors never predict it to perhaps be a gluten allergy. In most cases, the allergy tests performed never guarantee a 100% accurate result which is why my advice would be to do what I did. The hit and trial method works and is not only result based but also safer where you keep one ingredient in your diet while you eliminate another particular one to understand which ingredient is not suiting your body. I recently met someone who turns out is also gluten allergic but was completely unaware about it and shared her case with me. While she had no skin infection or blaring symptoms the way I did, she used to complain of serious migraines for years. She followed a healthy diet always but there was gluten present in that as well. But when she locked those gates and gluten from her diet, voila the migraines that had bothered her for years simply vanished.

It is a fact, that nearly 90% of those who avoid gluten because of an allergy factor or otherwise, notice an improved digestive function in the first week itself. It has now been over three years since I have been on a gluten free diet and the person I was before all this began is no more. Now if I ingest gluten by mistake, I can distinctly identify the signs which appear and immediately take care. I'm a new person today but my heart is still the same and does not miss out on anything it desires. The main reason for that is my better half who has always managed to find gluten free flour and several other products which are now available in Indian markets much more conveniently than before. Without her, my love with pizza would never have been requited and the void would have remained forever but fortunately not anymore. Even with a gluten free diet now I gorge on everything from breads to cakes to pastas, making sure they are prepared with special flour for me. Today, I live with a different perspective to life having faced a time where I had wished it would all just end.

The beginning of the end or the end of the beginning, you decide now.

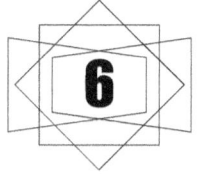

The Vocal Pacifier

The heart wants what the heart wants.

Those who understood, do it well and those who don't have yet to tell.

So it would come as no prime time surprise to the reader that as kids we all had our secrets. Our innocent summers would be full off fun and most of them included eating things we were otherwise always restricted to. The fondest memory I still have is of a neighbor who used to live downstairs and was the only woman who liked cats. Every year whenever there was a birthday in her family, she would distribute these delectable orange coloured candies which every kid got, two piece each. Several jaws would drop as my friends would notice I was the only one not eating the candy immediately and storing it in my pocket for later. I actually would do that to complete my duty of giving it to my parents as we were not allowed to eat any candy, chocolate or cold drink outside. Fair enough, except for the time my father in his steely response took it from me and just threw it in the garbage bag.

Just heartbreaking!

As a young elephant I hung on to my emotions but once we grew up we made up for all those times. We had a one point agenda: to try everything in life. Whether it was a cold drink hidden in my bag or a full stomach from eating chowmein or chocolate all afternoon, I played every card in the book and transcended from the innocent child to the naughty brat in five easy years. But somewhere my father was right as with most of these tempting delicacies and drinks come preservatives and artificial ingredients. Hence our throat being affected was a rather common symptom to observe but on every diagnosis my father would weave a meticulous recreation of how worse it could be if we did not pay attention.

The symptoms would come in many forms and could vary from pain in the throat, excessive sputum to irritation or continuous coughing. Judging on the gravity of the symptoms, my father would administer me Homeopathic medicine *Belladonna* and *Mercurious Solubilis* and assure me everything would be fine. His confidence would always make me marvel at him as a child but he would pull us back to remind us that we must gargle with warm water and salt. Nothing it seems could cure as expertly as a natural remedy and for me a problem with throat was always more dramatic as I would get a temperature if not treated soon. Don't be alarmed as there are others who face symptoms produced by same reasons such as sinus or sleepless nights due to cough. No doubt after gargling just twice and taking the Homeopathic medicine prescribed by my father, the turning point was evident and I felt better the next day itself.

I learnt very early in life never to lie to our doctor or our lawyer; they might just save our life. As years passed, my father's faith in Homeopathic and how he treated me when my throat did not feel right was further proof to substantiate the truth in it. Indeed I noticed, as a doctor my father was not in a practice of simply prescribing any medicine that would finish the job but his loyalty lay in finding a safer way with Homeopathy to cure it. It is not always easy as most people don't like to visit a doctor for something as small as a throat itch or a cough. They finally start getting serious when their throat is painful or not allowing them from eating their favourite papdi-chaat[5] anymore. Then there are patients who would never tell what they really ate while my father expertly but repeatedly kept asking them the same question. The truth can be diabolical as well as self-explanatory and I personally have never waited long enough to risk my health over it.

"Come on Somesh we are all going in to have dinner", my mom called me as we were at my cousin's wedding dinner in a posh hotel that night.

"Be right there, ma", came my instant response that could be mistook as a reflex. I required only sixty seconds being able to drown myself in as much cold drinks I wanted. The next day

---

[5] very popular Indian traditional street food.

the chilled cold drinks with ice caught up to me and I woke up feeling miserable. My throat was affected and that was translating to my nose feeling blocked as well. Judging the situation was getting aggravated faster than Homeopathy could treat; my father immediately put me on a five day course of antibiotic. This should not be misconstrued as after the antibiotic course my father treated me with Homeopathic medicine which took care of the remaining sinus and that prevented me from ever requiring a sinus operation. In the last two decades I have realized it is not impossible to get Homeopathic medicine but it is difficult certainly to change human nature. Most people tend to misjudge or undermine throat conditions until it gets worse. Even though all of us are taught during our school days how the throat is connected to the ear, for many the concept is absent when their bad throat translates into a serious sinus infection or asthma.

Like I said, those who understand it understand it well. One of my closest neighbor was a girl who studied in school with me and was the perfect partner when we were up to no good as kids. A true vagabond she was, fearless but loyal to whoever she called a friend. But we bonded also over our love for food and everything we saw in advertisements. In 2007, I spoke to her online as I was not in India and our conversation was rather mundane but a low toned one. She confided in me that she did not feel well and had a bad throat for which she has been prescribed antibiotics by her doctor.

"Wow that does not sound good! Please take care and I hope you are doing gargles", was my obvious reply to her.

"Yeah, yeah don't worry I'm having ice cream and I'm very happy", she replied. I was not surprised and actually believed her. She has always been an extremist and hated being told what to do so this nature of hers I was quite familiar with. We chatted a while longer and I signed off promising her to speak soon again. After one week, I got a call from my father who in a very serious tone informed me that my friend had passed away. Over the last few days her condition had worsened and doctors had to perform an emergency tonsillitis operation, which resulted in another complication and she was unable to make it. There are very few times in my life when I have been so overcome by grief that it made me completely numb, unable to react. This was one of those times.

Not only was she a beloved friend of mine who I had grown up with but to imagine her losing her life to an ailment which started from a pristine bad throat, made the loss very real for me. Till date I have not been able to fill the void left by her and there are loads more in the same vein. This unfortunate incident could have so easily been avoided that it made me realize how lightly people take such ailments without knowing what they can snowball into. Even then, I have come across a variety of educated illiterates who feel proud in boasting they have a cough since months and is a part of their family now since it doesn't bother them. What we don't realize is that having a bad throat over time can lead to other implications and in most cases Sinus, which itself is notorious for triggering a whole other world of symptoms. There is nothing to be proud of here; there is nothing to boast about.

Until 2019, whenever I wore a mask while stepping out, people gawked at me as if I was a patient released from the mental institute. There were others who laughed and deemed me to be a product of a typical "doctor's family" – overprotective and paranoid. This was even after me politely explaining that I was having a bad throat and simply did not want to give them my blessings in the form of a cough.

Being in one of the most highly polluted countries in the world, one would assume the attention would be more severe to such cases in our country. But for the society we live in, most questions are dismissed or met with a sharp rebuttal till the situation is very dire and the doctors are expected to fulfill the role of a God as well. The bemusing truth is that most people suffer coughs throughout the year and stop treating themselves. But for symptoms that arise early in case of a bad throat, I have witnessed Homeopathic medicines such as *Belladonna* and *Mercurious Solubilis* certainly work wonders. Not only do they argue their own case with evident results but actually help us in the new world that we are facing in today's time.

Our father has always taught us to live our life based on the famous English proverb, "a stitch in time, saves nine."

It is time we shared the benefits of our experiences with the world that we are today.

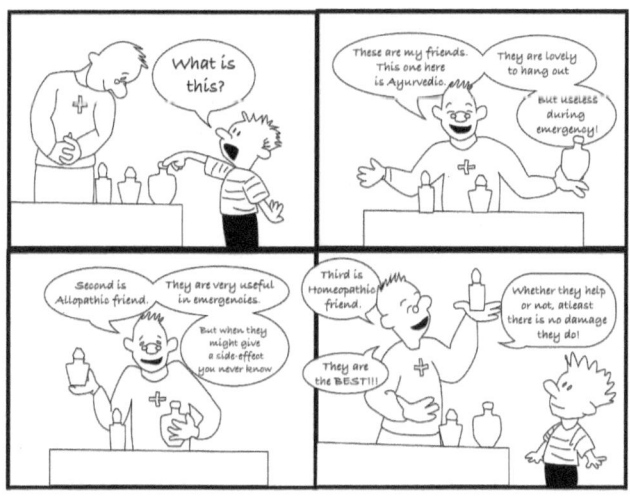

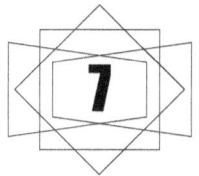

The Alpha Legacy

The world doesn't have a plan for a healthy future.

More than anything, the recent COVID pandemic in 2020 has showed us we are mere mortals when it comes to understanding how the human body is prone to getting affected by pathogens still foreign to man.

Let's face the grim truth, with climate change and air pollutants rising, the COVID pandemic is yet another blow risking the future of human existence. As more and more awake to these daunting on-goings, the medical experts are notably busy finding a cure. Human life they say will be safe again but never the same which is a fact hard to swallow for most of us.

We feel estranged from the social connect we had with the world and don't know what the future holds. Well the future holds whatever we make of it today by taking care of ourselves not just mentally but physically. Through the last two decades I have experienced firsthand the benefits of being treated with Homeopathy and pointed them out for the reader here. While there may not have seemed a reason strong enough before, over the course of time Homeopathy has saved me from other side-effects which are never underlined while being treated with Allopathic medicines. These side-effects at times can be worse than the disease itself.

The quality of a good life can have different meanings and it can never be defined by one element alone. A person with a six pack abs is not necessarily more fit than another who probably doesn't have a six pack to showoff but has a stronger immunity instead. This is one of the reasons why there is no hack to getting a healthier body by simply following one aspect alone. The composition is a mixture of a diet that your body deserves, paying attention to the real signals your body gives, regular exercises to keep the blood pumping and being aware about medications that are a part of our lives. The improvement is gradual but certainly a noticeable one and I write this as a bonafide speaker for Homeopathy today.

The world is still growing and it is essential for us to adapt and find methods that help the human body treat it with least or no side effects at all. With an open heart and an open mind, I am still learning the miracles and pitfalls of the medical arena as a patient. I encourage everyone who comes across my sphere to speak out and share their suffering as we are not alone. Now more than ever is the time that we share, learn and adapt with each other. Our story can make a difference to someone we have never probably heard of even. The only surreal fact I learnt about Homeopathy over decades was that it does its job silently without a murmur, but also functions in relation to the patient's characteristics.

Furthermore, one should not be fooled into believing that taking a high potency will guarantee relief sooner, which is not how Homeopathy functions. Prevention will always be better than cure and it makes complete sense to visit an expert professional when the symptoms do not subside or stop making sense entirely. Every sign we notice helps the doctor in better understanding our situation from a magnified point of view and confirming the culprit. Remember, there is no best doctor, only the right doctor.

There will be moments in your life where you will be overwhelmed by the power of making a decision for your own health and after reading my book, if you choose the right treatment that is safe for your body.

My work here is done.

www.ingramcontent.com/pod-product-compliance
Lightning Source LLC
Chambersburg PA
CBHW021018180526
45163CB00005B/2017